A Complete Guide to Weight Loss

JAMES DONOVAN, MD

CreateSpace Self-Publishing Platform
North Charleston, SC
LCCN: 2013909029
All Rights Reserved
ISBN-13: 978-1484133835
ISBN-10: 1484133838

© 2012

I would like to thank my many patients for giving me the incentive to complete this project. It has been their success in weight loss, disease modification, and life transformation that leads me to believe this plan is something that can work for anyone. Just today I had a patient tell me he gave away his CPAP machine because he is never going to get fat again. The long term success these patients have had makes me feel like a better person, and I hope you will, too.

I ask all my patients at goal weight if they think they are the same people they were when we met, and they all say no. I guess you cannot be the same person and keep your weight off. My goal is to change the way you relate to food. And when you do, we'll both have changed – for good.

I really must thank my mother-in-law, Marianne Nold. Not just for putting up with me as her "favorite son-in-law" (I am her only son-in-law) for these last 25 years, but for spending those many hours on the phone and home alone editing this work. It was her expertise that turned my archaic writing into something more easily read. Thank you, Marianne; you are my favorite mother-in-law too!

Table of Contents

Chapter 1	Introduction	p. 4
Chapter 2	Feast and Famine	p. 6
Chapter 3	Metabolic Window	p. 8
Chapter 4	The Insulin Response	p. 12
Chapter 5	Why Fight Genetics?	P. 16
Chapter 6	The Equation for Life	p. 21
Chapter 7	Glycemic Index	p. 23
Chapter 8	Becoming a Successful Loser	p. 33
Chapter 9	Why We Look Like a Food Pyramid	p. 37
Chapter 10	The Measuring Cup Free Diet	p. 49
Chapter 11	Metabolic Syndrome Work-up	p. 70
Conclusion		p. 75

Chapter 1
Introduction

My mission in the field of weight loss began about five years ago when I was camping with my wife's family. While we were at the beach it occurred to me that her relatives are all naturally thin people while my family is naturally fat. In college I raced bicycles and did triathlons. At that time I was in great shape - 4% body fat. I even remember thinking I should weigh a little more because I was tiring out after 70 miles of biking, and I needed a little more reserve. Then I got married, went to medical school, and had two kids - a stressful life. I had every excuse for weight gain covered. Well, both my wife and I had extra pounds, me about 80 more than when we met and my wife about 30. Not only that, my pictures looked just like my grandfather's. To me it was destiny.

My wife, however, did not have the same excuses. Her family was all naturally thin. We were doing something very wrong. I had ideas, but no plan. Around the same time I noted this, my sister fell off a ladder and injured her knee. Her doctor told her that without weight loss she was looking at a knee replacement in her forties. She joined LA Weight Loss and had excellent results. About then, LA Weight Loss opened in our town, so against my wife's protestations we both went for a consultation. Desperate times called for desperate measures. We did it. We both lost about 30 pounds. My wife was amazed at how easy it was. She wasn't even trying that hard. Her weight flew off, and she was a poster child for weight loss. Me - well, that was a different story. I fought for every pound I lost. I still do. It was obvious to me that there was a profound difference in our genetics, how we respond to food and dieting, and our will power to lose weight. Not only that, I had a real knack for cheating on a restricted diet that my wife didn't feel. It wasn't that I wanted to cheat. I knew the consequences; I just would lose control. I was stress eating - whether from fatigue, frustration, or just a hard day. I am a physician. I can study for 16 hours at a crack. I can sit in a deer stand quiet as a mouse for hours on end, but I have a hard time controlling eating. It wasn't compulsive eating; it was craving. I had to find out what was going on.

    I learned a lot at LA Weight Loss and had become inspired. In my practice I started to work with my obese patients on weight loss. First, I would send them to dieticians - with little to no success. Then I would talk to them about what I did, and that helped some. But I had to do better. I went to a couple of conferences on obesity - some good, some bad. Then I discovered the American Society for Bariatric Physicians (ASBP), and that is where I learned what no one else had been able to explain to me. This group of doctors understands obesity and knows how to achieve weight loss. More importantly, they understand adiposopathy - the disease of excess fat. Identified by Dr Harold Bays MD, adiposopathy treats obesity as a chronic disease just like heart disease and diabetes. The difference, however, is that obesity doesn't cause injury to just one organ such as the heart or kidney. It affects all of them.

This booklet is a summary of the two-hour lecture I give to all of my obesity patients before they start working with me. We spend two hours in a group session because knowledge is power, and you need a lot of power to fight obesity. I want people to change the way they relate to food. This takes time. Studies show that if you can lose weight and keep it off for two years you have about an 85% chance of keeping it off for a lifetime. Why is this important? Because obesity makes all diseases worse. For example, a 20-pound weight gain for a woman between ages 20 and midlife doubles her risk for breast cancer. The number one modifiable risk for breast cancer is weight gain, and no one is talking about it. Excess fat causes the disease of adiposopathy.

Chapter 2
Feast and Famine

Depending on whom you read and what you believe, we Homo sapiens (the smart apes) have been on this planet for about 100,000 years in our present form. About every seven years we have undergone regional droughts and famines. The Bible even has a story about Joseph predicting that the Egyptians would have seven years of plenty followed by seven years of famine. For all of our history, except the last 60 or so years, we have fought famine. Here in the USA, our last significant experience of it was during the Dust Bowl years. Since then, transportation and refrigeration have saved us from the problems still facing many parts of the world today.

Also, in the last 40 years we have seen a radical change in the American diet. We have been told to eat a low fat, high carbohydrate diet (remember the traditional food pyramid). In addition, fast foods and convenience foods at the grocery store have led to a diet much different than what our grandparents ate.

We love our fast food restaurants, too. We eat lots of fast food, and why shouldn't we? It is cheap, convenient, and it tastes good. There are three things we seek in our diet at a visceral level: salt, sugar, and fat. Fast food delivers these in spades. The restaurant industry has learned what we want so well that, to compete for our business, they have greatly increased our serving sizes to a point that would make a person from the 1940s swoon. They can do this because for the first time in human history food is cheap to produce. However, the cost we are actually paying is staggering. Because of the obesity epidemic, which is now world-wide, we have the first generation of children in the US who will not live as long as their parents. This is a sobering thought. So why does it happen, and what can we do about it?

Chapter 3
Metabolic Window

When we are maintaining a stable weight we are at a metabolic set point. We can eat a little more or a little less and still tend to maintain our weight within a few pounds. But there is controversy in the literature about the validity of a set point. We may come to this point because our weight catches up with our eating habits. This controversy is valid in that people who weigh more need more calories than people who weigh less. The question is do we who eat more than we need gain weight up to the point where our energy use matches our intake? For example, does a person weigh 300 pounds because he eats enough for a three hundred pound person? Or is his weight predetermined by his hypothalamus in his brain? Regardless of the academic arguments, we all know that we can eat a little more or less and we won't lose or gain any significant weight. I like to think of this as more of a window than set point. We gain a little weight or lose a little weight, but we don't seem to go out of our window. Most people fluctuate about 5-10 pounds within this window.

Nevertheless, we get tired of our extra weight. So we

go on a diet. We lose about 20 pounds, and now we need less energy. Because our metabolic window does not change with our weight change, we move higher into our metabolic window.

Now we need to eat a lot less to lose more weight but eat very little more to regain our lost weight. It gets frustrating to lose any more weight. We decide that this is a good new weight for us. So what do we do? We go "off our diet." What this usually means is that we stop eating less because we are happy with our weight loss, and we return to our old eating habits. We eat what we did at the old higher weight; and, since our bodies need less to function, we store that extra energy we don't need as fat and gain the weight back. Usually, though, we don't just gain the weight back. We add a couple more pounds to what we weighed before the weight loss. Before long we are dieting again – the yo-yo diet.

Why does this happen? As far as your body knows you just went through a famine. You don't think so because food was all around you, but your stomach doesn't see it that way. You lost all of the weight by going for your reserves (stored fat), and when the diet-famine was over your body did what it had to do - replenish its losses. Not only that, but it thought, "That was a close one! Better make sure we have a little more for next time!" By now you have gained a couple of extra pounds.

Whether this is because of set points or metabolic

windows is certainly controversial and difficult to prove. Do we eat a habitual amount of food so that our weight will naturally center because of the mechanics and physics of energy expenditure, or is there a mechanism in our hypothalamus that desires a specified weight? No one knows for sure. I think it makes sense from an evolutionary standpoint to consider the following example.

Imagine 100,000 years ago when we were chasing rabbits to survive. We live in a beautiful valley with plenty of fruit in the trees, vegetables on the ground, and rabbits everywhere. Here in a proverbial Garden of Eden we do not need to work very hard to get our food. We are fat, dumb, and happy, but we are also human. We constantly look at the mountains around us and wonder what is on the other side. So one day we pack our things, climb over the mountain, come down the other side, and what do we find? A tropical beach. White sands are greeted by a warm, turquoise sea while palm trees provide shade under an equatorial sun. There are fish plentiful in the sea and coconuts and breadfruit ripe for picking. We were right; the grass is definitely greener on the other side of the hill. The weather is hot and we just aren't as hungry. We lose weight. We look good.

Yet, there is a problem. All of us who have lost significant weight in the past know what this is. It is a small panic. It isn't conscious. A fear from deep within that something bad is going to happen with this weight loss - we are going to starve. We have a deep-seated fear that famine will come here, too. It has happened throughout human history. We have to get back to where it was safe. We need to gain the weight we lost. We need to go back where we know the food source is sound and predictable. So we climb back over the mountain and away from our tropical paradise.

As sad as this may seem, it has made us who we are. We do not want to starve in a famine. We who have a weight problem come from a long line of people with an evolutionary advantage culled over years of feast and famine. We are gifted energy storers. While the thin among us say it is a willpower issue, they are only partly correct. We do have a willpower problem keeping weight off, but our battle with willpower is not as simple as the naturally thin would like to believe. We are designed to store energy as our ancestors did. To look down one's nose at an obese person is like a gazelle looking down its nose at a dog that lives in a butcher shop and thinking the dog just has no will power. Certainly, willpower plays a role but more is involved than what any naturally thin person or gazelle might imagine.

There is a group of people who, when eating, display three characteristics: lack of satiety (feeling full), obsessing over food, and loss of control. These symptoms are seen in both thin and obese people. To give an idea of what this is like I will describe myself. I can be in a car with a full bag of Doritos. If I have one, I will eat until the chips are gone - even after they no longer taste good. If I put them in the back seat, I know they are there and will likely go for them again. If I do not have any, it's not a problem. If I start eating, then I can experience all three characteristics. Does this happen every time? No, but on a long trip with no distractions and factors such as fatigue and boredom, it can be a challenge. I used to think everyone was like this. Well, a lot of people are not. Not my wife and not the people who aren't reading this booklet.

In people, thin or fat, who display these symptoms – lack of satiety, obsessing over food, losing control – brain studies show that eating carbohydrates and fats such as Doritos stimulates the amygdala (our brain's center of pleasure and reward) in a way similar to that of heroin or cocaine in drug addicts. Thus, for a thin person to say we have a problem with willpower is like saying a heroin addict's problem is just a lack of willpower. There is no question that it takes a tremendous amount of willpower for a drug addict to come clean, but to ignore the physiology is folly.

Losing weight takes willpower – lots of it. But understanding the science can help.

Chapter 4
The Insulin Response

Why do some people gain weight and others do not? I have a good friend and hunting buddy I will call Dave because that is his name. Dave is one of those naturally thin people. Sure, he is a busy, hyper sort of guy, but so am I when I have had enough rest. One fine summer day I was walking my dog around the neighborhood at about 4 PM and came to Dave's house. He was working in his garage as he often does, so I stopped by for a chat. His wife was there, who, like me, struggles with weight. As we were talking he suddenly drew a blank face and then said that he had forgotten to eat lunch that day. All he had eaten was a jelly doughnut at 8 AM. He said to me, "Don't you hate it when you forget to eat?" I looked at his wife, she looked at me, and we laughed. We never forget to eat! In fact, his wife said that come fall while deer hunting I could shoot him for that comment, and she wouldn't tell a soul (she was kidding). While that may seem extreme, it raises two points. First, we naturally gifted storers are quite sensitive about our weight; and secondly, don't tick off your wife with comments like that. However, it got me thinking. Why are he and I so different? It comes down to insulin.

    Whatever you know about insulin, I want you to understand that insulin's primary job is not to regulate blood sugar. Insulin's main job is as an energy storage hormone. Sugar, or glucose, is the molecule of energy exchange in our bodies. We burn glucose because it is a very efficient molecule, easily soluble in our tissues, and it carries a lot of energy in its chemical bonds. We can burn protein and fats, but our bodies like sugar because it is so efficient.

Our bodies also love homeostasis. That is, our bodies want everything to be in balance. Our blood sugars need to be in a certain range for optimum function. When our blood sugars begin to rise, we release insulin to drive glucose (sugar) into our cells and return our blood sugars to their normal range. The picture is more understandable when we see what insulin does. Before we eat, our blood sugar is in check. The liver has its own store of glucose called glycogen, and sugar is released from the liver to keep our sugar level up. If we are out of our glycogen stores, the liver can even manufacture about 90% of our needs with the kidney making the rest. We do not need to get glucose through our diet. After we eat, assuming we are not expending energy hiking or running, we do not immediately need this energy. As our blood sugar rises, our pancreas releases insulin because we have more energy than we need. Insulin then drives that sugar into many tissues, and what is left over goes into fat to be stored as energy because calories are very precious and we do not waste them. When we eat more food energy than we need, we don't sweat it out, poop it out, pee it out, or breathe it out. We either use it, or we store it. For the first 100,000 years our ancestors were on this planet they worked too hard to get those calories and did not waste them. Today we have easy access to calories, and we store lots of them.

So what happens to Dave when he eats a jelly

doughnut at 8 AM? As he digests the doughnut he releases insulin to combat the rising blood sugar, and his insulin levels follow the blood sugar rise, decreasing as his blood sugar decreases. His liver releases stored sugar as needed, and he can go all day on that one doughnut. He is efficient, and he is thin. When his wife and I eat a jelly doughnut at 8 AM, we release insulin just like he did; however, we release a lot of insulin. Our pancreas acts as if it's in a panic and doesn't want to lose one calorie. We drive that sugar into our fat cells as quickly as we can. About two hours later we are starving. Our blood sugars are now too low. We want another doughnut (I actually want Snickers) because the extra insulin we release was more than we needed for homeostasis and our blood sugar dropped too low. This is a very efficient way to store energy. Lions do this. They gorge on the wildebeest until they cannot eat any more then lie down in the shade. About two hours later when their stomachs are empty and their blood sugar drops, they get up and eat some more. They need to store as much as they can because their meals are not regular or predictable. Americans do something similar on Thanksgiving. We gorge ourselves on turkey, potatoes, corn, stuffing, and dessert – let's be honest, desserts. Then we lie down, watch the Detroit Lions get beat, and about two hours later (at halftime) we get up for the leftovers and gorge ourselves again. At least now we will make it through winter.

You can test yourself. Have a nice plate of pancakes

and see how you feel a couple of hours later. If you are really hungry, you are one of us. In fact, I can get woozy and sweaty and mildly confused. This is actually a hypoglycemic episode similar to what diabetics with too much insulin experience and is called an insulin reaction or diabetic reaction. For non-diabetics it is called reactive hypoglycemia. While I do not have diabetes, we who have reactive hypoglycemia are at increased risk of diabetes because of our exaggerated insulin response.

We know that obesity has a strong genetic component, and now we understand some of the physiology. So, why fight it? Well, 100,000 years ago we wouldn't have to fight it. We were lucky to live to 40 years old. Now we live twice as long, and that's where the double-edged sword of obesity hits us hard.

Chapter 5
Why Fight Genetics?

We define Relative Risk (RR) as the disease risk of a person with a certain characteristic compared to a person without that characteristic. The one without the characteristic is considered to have an RR of one. We will call this control person a thin fit person, defined as a person of normal weight (body mass index of 18.5-25) who walks 2000 steps or about one mile a day. If you are obese (BMI of 30 or more) and unfit, you have a relative risk of death and disease of about eight. This means you have eight times the risk of a thin fit person to develop the diseases most often associated with obesity - diabetes, heart attack, and stroke.

If you lose 10% of your weight, such as going from 200 pounds to 180 pounds, you can reduce your risk of death and disease by 50% - RR 8 to 4. While you are still at four times the risk of a thin fit person, you cut your current risk in half. Let's put that into perspective. If you come to me as a patient with hyperlipidemia (high cholesterol) and I put you on a statin (Lipitor, Zocor or the like) and get your cholesterol down to goal, I can lower your risk of heart attack by about 38%. If I can just get you to reduce your weight 10%, it cuts your risk 50%. This far outweighs the effect of medication alone. This is one very important reason that as a family physician I became involved in bariatric medicine. Weight loss is the single most effective modifiable reducer of disease for human beings on earth today.

So what happens with another 10% weight loss? Your relative risk of death and disease is reduced another 10%. That is right. Every 10% weight loss after the first 10% reduces your risk by an additional 10%. The point is that while losing weight and getting to a normal weight would be ideal, if one can just lose 10%, his or her risk is cut in half. On a societal level, imagine reducing diabetes, heart attack, and stroke by 50%. Healthcare costs would plummet.

If fact, obesity does more than contribute to diabetes, heart attack, and stroke. Remember, a woman who gains 20 pounds between age 18 and mid life doubles her risk for breast cancer. Why is no one talking about it? Because weight loss is the hardest thing a physician can motivate patients to do. But it doesn't have to be.

Just 10% weight loss will improve of all the diseases listed below:

- Heart disorders
- Hypertension
- Impaired immunity
- Impaired respiratory function
- Infection following wounds
- Liver disease
- Low back pain
- OB/GYN complications
- Pain
- Asthma
- Sleep apnea
- Stroke
- Surgical complications
- Urinary stress incontinence
- Osteoarthritis
- Rheumatoid Arthritis
- Neural tube defects of babies
- Cancer of the breast, esophagus, stomach, colon, endometrium, and kidney
- Coronary artery disease
- Carpal tunnel syndrome
- Chronic venous insufficiency

- Daytime sleepiness
- Blood clots
- Diabetes type II
- Kidney disease
- Gall bladder disease
- Pancreatitis
- Gout

Included in this list are the usual suspects such as heart disease, diabetes, and stroke, but there are also inflammatory diseases such as rheumatoid arthritis and infections. This is because fat, in particular visceral fat, the fat around your abdominal organs, is very hormonally active. Most of these hormones, such as interlukin-1 and tumor necrosis factor, are inflammatory and harmful. We now know that visceral fat produces over 100 adipokines or fat hormones. This is why fat is involved in worsening your prognosis with cancers, blood clots, wound healing, and complications of pregnancy.

Obesity, like heart disease, diabetes, and asthma, is a chronic disease. It cannot be cured, only controlled. Fortunately, there is hope. Remember, if a person loses weight and keeps it off for two years, there is an 85% chance the weight will stay off. If I could prescribe a medication for hypertension for two years that would give you an 85% chance of reducing your blood pressure for the rest of your life, would you take it? How about if I told you the side effects would be more energy, better sleep, better self-esteem, and a reduction in all other health problems? Weight loss can do it. The problem most physicians have with weight loss is that they do not have the education or the time to help patients with this chronic disease. So how do you do it?

Chapter 6
The Equation for Life

Let's begin with what I call the equation for life:

$$T_{EE} = BMR + A_{EE} + NEAT$$

T_{EE} = Total energy expenditure

BMR = Basal Metabolic Rate (the energy to keep one's temperature at 98.6^0)

A_{EE} = Active Energy Expenditure (energy used in an exercise program)

NEAT = Non-Exercise Activities of Thermogenesis (energy use for all daily activities)

Putting values to this equation will show us how to lose weight. Total energy expenditure (T_{EE}) is all the calories we burn in a day and is set at 100%. This does not include any extra calories we take in and don't use. The Basal Metabolic Rate (BMR) is the fixed energy expenditure we possess, which is different for everybody. BMR is the energy used to keep the system running (think $98.6°$) and includes the 10% calorie loss used to digest our food. BMR is equal to about 60-80% of all the calories used in a day. Active Energy Expenditure (A_{EE}) is 0% if no exercise is performed; and, for the average person, a good workout can lead to about 10% calorie expenditure. This leaves Non-Exercise Activities of Thermogenesis (NEAT) to fill in the gaps, thus, 10-40% of calories burned. Therefore the equation looks like this:

$$T_{EE} = BMR + A_{EE} + NEAT$$
$$100\% = (60 \text{ to } 80\%) + (0 \text{ to } 10\%) + (10 \text{ to } 40\%)$$

By studying this equation we can see that most of the calories we use in a day are fixed in our BMR. If we really work hard, we can burn up to 10% of our calories. By doing little extras in our day, such as walking a little more, we can consume up to 40% more calories than by just being sedentary. The most important point of this equation shows us that it is not exercise that will lead us to weight loss because all the energy burned is only up to 10% for the average person. Calorie restriction is the key. Most of our calorie expenditure each day is fixed in just keeping us warm. If most of the calories used cannot be changed (except through the use of chemicals to speed metabolism – not recommended), then calorie restriction will cause the most efficient weight loss.

While I am certainly a fan of exercise because of its protective benefits to our health and well-being, it is not the cornerstone of weight loss. Think of exercise as a benefit from weight loss. You will find that as you lose weight, you will want to exercise. Right now at 20, 30, 40, 60 or more pounds overweight, you are exercising just by moving this weight. To show that being obese is exercise, I encourage you to go to the grocery store and carry an additional five pound bag of flour around for every five pounds you lose. As you lose the weight, you will see how much exercise being fat really involves.

That is it - all we need to know. To lose weight we need to eat less than what we burn. We have discussed why we are fat, why we should lose weight, and how to lose weight. Now we will learn about the keys to metabolism that we can manipulate for maximum weight loss.

Chapter 7
Glycemic Index

An excellent experiment performed by Dr. David Jenkins of the University of Toronto paved the way for us to manipulate our diet for maximum fat loss. He and his researchers identified two groups of people we'll call group A and group B. First, they matched them as best they could. These groups were matched not just by height and weight, but also through metabolic testing so that they were identical in energy processing abilities; that is, they were two metabolically equivalent groups. Then both groups were fed a 1000-calorie diet. I am here to tell you that if you are bigger than a child, you need more than 1000 calories a day to maintain your weight. These people were certain to lose weight on this diet. The third thing they did was to make sure that both groups had adequate protein to maintain a positive nitrogen balance. By insuring they had adequate protein in their diet they inhibited the loss of lean body mass (muscles and organs). If you recall, back in the late 1970s and 1980s, a liquid protein diet was very popular. It was well marketed but not well thought out. The person who designed this diet did not use a complete protein in his drink. Of the 20 or so amino acids our bodies use to make proteins, we need about eight in our diet that our bodies cannot make. These are the essential amino acids and must be consumed in order for us to stay healthy. Because this diet did not include all of these amino acids, some people became sick and some died. Dr. Jenkins and his team were aware of this and made sure their subjects had proper protein.

    To make up the rest of the 1000 daily calories, Dr. Jenkins added sugars to the protein drinks he had made. Group A was given simple sugars such as those found in table sugar and white bread. Group B was given complex sugars such as those found more in fruits and vegetables. This study ran for about 12 weeks.

    After 12 weeks of the protein drink diet, the researchers looked at the results. They were not too surprised to find that both groups had lost weight because they were on calorie restricted diets. However, group B on the complex sugar diet lost more weight than group A on the simple sugar diet. Not only that, but Group A lost a significantly larger amount of lean body mass (muscles and organs) than group B. So here we have two groups on the same calorie diet, with the same protein and micronutrients but different sugars, showing significant differences in not only the amount of weight lost but also in the kind of weight lost. These groups were matched metabolically, so if a calorie were a calorie, they both should have lost the same amount and the same kind of weight, but they did not.

Out of this research came a term many of us have heard - glycemic index. Glycemic index is the measure of how much insulin is released in response to a specific food intake. The glycemic index concept spawned two very successful diets, the South Beach Diet and the Zone Diet. Both of these diets take advantage of our body's own hormonal underpinnings to maximize fat loss while minimizing lean mass loss. LA Weight Loss also uses this very successfully. Weight Watchers has recently recognized this and now is assigning different points based on the glycemic index of foods.

Why is glycemic index important? Again, it boils down to insulin. As discussed earlier, insulin's main purpose is not the regulation of blood sugar; rather, insulin is released under periods of excess energy in the blood stream (as glucose) to drive this extra energy into the cells. In our case, this means that insulin is a prime driver of fat deposition. (Okay, we often eat too much, too.) Here it should be noted that fat people do eat more than thin people, but not much more. In fact, obese people eat about 200 calories more than thin people each day. Divided among three meals, that is only about 70 calories per meal or less than one slice of bread or one more snack a day than a thin person. The problem is that when an extra 200 calories is multiplied by 365 days a year it equals an extra 20.8 pounds of calories a year. Fortunately, we do have a metabolic window that usually prevents us from gaining that much weight.

To understand insulin better, first imagine you are sitting in a chair reading a book. You get the idea to have a doughnut. You eat the doughnut and sit down to read your book again. There has been no change in energy needs, just energy consumption. As the doughnut is digested, the sugar is absorbed into the blood stream. Because our bodies want equilibrium, the pancreas releases insulin to drive this extra energy into the cells. The truth is, when you eat a calorie you either use it or store it. Energy is too precious to waste. Historically, it has always been too hard to come by calories to waste even one.

Keep this in mind as we look at insulin's effect on three main tissues of the body: muscle, liver, and fat.

The first tissue we will consider is skeletal muscle.

During a fasting state, skeletal muscle primarily uses triglycerides for energy. When a sugary meal is eaten and insulin is released, the stimulation of the insulin receptors on the muscle cell causes the muscle to absorb glucose, and the skeletal muscle will immediately convert to using sugar for energy. This causes a build-up of triglycerides in the muscle, which eventually spill into the blood stream and cause triglycerides to become elevated. (I am purposely leaving out a lot of biochemistry.) This is why people with high blood sugars or high insulin levels (insulin resistance) tend to have high triglycerides.

Muscle cells are interesting in that they will also store some glucose for instant energy. This is important because if you are walking through the jungle and a lion jumps out in your path or crossing the street and a speeding car runs a stop sign, you need instant energy for the fight or flight reflex. This store of glucose allows for that.

The second tissue to examine is the liver. The liver is an amazing organ. It is the only organ that will grow back if half is removed. It has many functions, but let's focus on what the liver does when stimulated by insulin.

The first thing the liver will do is store glucose in long loose chains called glycogen. We have about a 36-hour supply of glucose in the form of glycogen stored in our livers. Glucose acts like salt in that it has an osmotic effect. Just as salt makes you retain water, glucose retains water also. Thus, with this storage of glucose we also have stored extra water. We are a little like camels.

Imagine you are in the desert, and your car breaks down. To survive you have to walk out. In your liver you have a snack bar of glucose and a water supply to help you through this time. It is a great survival mechanism. It is also why, when we go on a diet, we first lose all of that "water weight." It's our liver using up the glucose and the water being washed away.

This brings me to a side bar. I was watching one of those shows on a learning channel about the super obese. It included an interview of a very heavy woman. She said something to the effect that she doesn't eat when she is hungry. I thought that was obvious, but then she said nobody in America does either. She hit the nail on the head. Now we have all been on diets that go well for three or four days. We lose all of our water weight, \ we are down 5-10 pounds, and we are excited. But then what happens? We get really hungry and we eat doughnuts. Why? Well, we have burned all of our sugar out of our liver, and now we need to switch our metabolism over to burning fats. This is a process that takes time. So our bodies do two things: first, we start burning more protein because it is relatively easy to do; second, we get hungry, truly hungry. We crave sugar, high energy foods, because we do not want to burn fat. Fat is for survival in a famine. Hunger is the drive to make sure there is nothing to eat before we break into our fat stores. This is the hunger the woman was talking about. This is true hunger. We don't let ourselves get to this point because we eat three or four times a day. We are never really hungry. She was right.

Bariatric surgeons take advantage of this system. If you have known anyone to have bariatric surgery (stomach staple, lap-band), they will tell you the surgeon put them on a two-week protein shake diet. Why? It is not because surgeons are cruel. It is because they want to shrink the liver. The liver sits right over the area of the gut where they want to work. By voiding the liver of glycogen and water, the liver may shrink 20%. This gives them much more room to work.

The liver is also able to manufacture glucose. Our brains function exclusively on glucose, using about 6 grams per hour. However, if we do not get sugar in our diet, the liver is able to make about 10 grams per hour and slows down to about 6 grams per hour during a prolonged starvation. This guarantees the brain its need for glucose. So we do not need carbohydrate in our diet; we can make what we need.

Insulin stimulates the liver to make cholesterol as well. This is one of the reasons why many obese people have elevated cholesterol. Not all, because there are many genetic factors that also influence cholesterol production. But if a person is obese, chances are he or she has elevated cholesterol or is being treated for high cholesterol.

Often if I see a patient who has elevated cholesterol, I

will recheck it at 10% weight loss. It is amazing how often the lipid profile will show dramatic improvement. (Remember a 10% weight loss has the biggest impact on your health.) This proves how significant an impact obesity and an obesity-inducing diet can have on cholesterol production.

Finally, insulin induces the storage of fat in the liver. Obese people tend to have fatty livers because the liver is a good place to store some fat. However, not a lot. When the liver stores enough fat to interrupt normal liver function, a condition called **non-alcoholic steatohepatitis** or NASH can develop. What NASH means is that the liver is inflamed, and it was caused by fat, not alcohol, the most common way to irritate a liver. This inflammatory condition caused by fat can result in liver failure. When obese people develop NASH it is a serious problem. Two treatments can solve this: weight loss and liver transplant. Reducing the fat load of the liver will resolve NASH because it is the inflammatory hormones produced by fat that are injuring the liver. Reduce the fat load, and the inflammatory hormones go away.

The third tissue to consider is adipose or fat. Of all of the ideas discussed in this work, the impact of insulin on fat cells is the single most important lesson. Remember, insulin's job in our body is not to manage our blood sugars; insulin is an energy storage hormone. Glucose is the currency of energy exchange in our bodies. It is a very efficient currency as it is easily absorbed, readily soluble in water, and packed with energy. When insulin is released in response to a rise in blood glucose, it is a lot like a trip to the grocery store.

Picture yourself at the grocery store. As you wander the aisles and gather the food on your list, you note a hunger stemming from all of the external food cues you encounter. (Grocers know what makes us tick.) So here you are - hungry with a cart full of groceries. Wisely, you decide, "I am not going to get a pack of doughnuts and eat them on the way home. I am going to make something at home." So you gather the goods and head home. Once there, you unload the car and put all of the groceries on the counter. You decide you cannot wait any longer. At this point, you are not going to go into the pantry and pull out the ingredients for a homemade hot dish; rather, you are going to eat the stuff in front of you on the counter. Our bodies are no different. If our bodies are in a state where there is extra energy floating in our blood stream (groceries on the counter) and the pancreas releases insulin in response, we do not want to burn our stored energy (ingredients in the pantry) because that is there for the next famine, which our genetics predict will happen as it always has.

When insulin binds to an adipocyte (fat cell), it causes two things. First, it causes the uptake of glucose into the cell and its conversion to fat for long-term storage. Remember, we do not want to waste a calorie, and if we are not going to use it now we will save it for potential bad times ahead.

Insulin's second significant role is that it inhibits the breakdown of fat for energy. Just as you do not want to go into the pantry to make a hot dish when the there is food on the counter, our bodies do not want to mobilize fat for energy when we have extra energy available in our blood stream. While there are many reasons for the obesity epidemic in America and the world, the change from a higher fat diet to a diet lower in fat (although we still eat a lot of fat) necessitated we get our calories from high carbohydrate sources. We went from a diet with low insulin stimulation to a diet with high insulin stimulation. This is no problem in itself if we eat a low enough calorie diet to use the fat we have, but we all eat more calories than our grandparents did. Insulin is doing its job by storing that energy and keeping us from mobilizing our fat in anticipation of coming famine.

In Dr. Jenkins' study, group A had a high-sugar, high-glycemic index diet. The researchers were causing the people in group A to have higher insulin levels even though they were on a low calorie diet. Because they needed more than 1000 calories a day for their bodily functions, the energy had to come from somewhere. Their fat cells were being told that there was enough energy so they held onto the fat. The body then needed to go elsewhere for energy, so it started to break down lean body mass. Thus, people in group A lost more lean body weight than people in group B. The people in group B fared much better. They were in need of extra energy just like group A, but because their insulin levels were much lower the adipose tissue (fat) was able to mobilize fat for energy. They were able to use the stored fat for the famine they were in, just as our bodies are designed to do.

Remember, when we have sugar in our blood, and insulin is released to drive it into the cells, insulin is also inhibiting us from mobilizing our fat for energy. This is what the glycemic index of food tells us. A food low in glycemic index causes little or no insulin release and allows us to use fat for energy. A food with a high glycemic index causes significant insulin release and inhibits us from mobilizing fat. We want to lose excess fat. To do so, we must be able to mobilize and use our fat stores. Therefore, we need to design an eating style that allows this to happen. I propose a three-pronged approach - reduce calorie intake, eat low glycemic index foods, and choose good quality protein.

Now we can look at how to keep weight off.

Chapter 8
Becoming a Successful Loser

How does one become a successful loser? An even hotter topic in bariatric medicine than how to get patients to lose weight is how to keep it off. Psychologists tell us it takes about 6-8 weeks to change a behavior and one to two years to make the new behavior permanent. Bariatric medicine tells us that if one loses weight and keeps it off for 1-2 years, there is an 85% chance of keeping it off for a lifetime. So how does this happen? How do we keep off the weight we worked so hard to lose?

The National Weight Control Registry is a national web site and on-going research project. It is a self-reporting survey of the strategies people use to keep their weight off. To qualify for this study one has to meet two main criteria. First, lose a minimum of thirty pounds; and second, keep it off for one year. This meets the criteria for behavior change outlined above. Amazingly, the average person on this registry has lost 60 pounds and kept it off for 5 years. These are truly successful losers. I encourage you to check out the web site (http://www.nwcr.ws/). You will be amazed at the amount of information available to you.

So how are they doing it? The answer is exercise - but not just some exercise. These people are doing an average of 60 minutes of activity a day they did not do before they lost weight. I suspect you think like I do - that you just don't have time for an hour of exercise every day. Well, neither do they. If you read my statement carefully, you will notice I said they are doing 60 minutes of <u>activity</u> they did not do before weight loss. This means at that at day's end they are not watching the same amount of TV. They are taking walks, even going to a gym, playing with kids, essentially doing all the things we want to do but can't because we are so heavy. If you take a

60-pound pack off your back, you will have more energy. You will not want to sit and watch 3-4 hours of TV a night while snacking. You will want to move – because you **can**.

Exercise is vital to weight loss. When people lose 10% of their weight, they also drop their metabolism by almost the same amount. Since we are about 75% water I like to think of the body as a big barrel of water. The barrel needs to be 98.6 degrees, so we light a fire underneath it. If I take out 10% of the water, I need less fire to get the water warm.

Another way to think about it is to look at the metabolic window idea. When we lose weight we move up in the metabolic window. Our bodies want us to put the weight back on so we will be ready for the next famine, like the one we were just in that we called a diet. The average difference in calorie needs for a person with a 10% weight loss is about 300-500 calories a day. This means you need 300-500 fewer calories a day to heat your water tank or 300-500 fewer calories a day to get back to the middle of your metabolic window.

When we walk, we burn about 100 calories for every mile we walk (figure about 100 yards per M&M). It takes the average person about 20 minutes to walk one mile. Thus, the people on the National Weight Control Registry who do 60 minutes of activity a day are burning about 300 more calories a day, or walking about three miles a day that they were not covering before weight loss. Again, for the average person, it takes about 2,000 steps to walk one mile. So to do 60 minutes a day, one has to walk about 6,000 more steps a day. This is very easy to measure. For about $10 you can buy a good pedometer that will count your steps for you. Put it on your belt in the morning and look at it at bedtime. Keep track as you lose weight, and you will be amazed at what weight loss does to your daily movement. Now, if you think, "This will not work for me as I am running at 110% all day, and there is no way I could get 6,000 more steps into my day," I say, "Hogwash!" The average New Yorker walks 10,000 steps a day. There are 24 hours a day in New York and 24 hours in your day (although it's said the New York minute is faster). It is easier for New Yorkers because they walk nearly everywhere they go. We drive everywhere we go. Even our malls are set up so we don't have to walk as far. To get our activity in we need NEAT (Non Exercise Activities of Thermogenesis). Carry each grocery bag by itself; carry several small loads of laundry one at a time; park in the last spot at the parking lot. Ever notice how those guys with the midlife crisis and the $50,000 sports cars parked sideways at the end of the lot are all thin? (and bald and wear too much jewelry?) Each little step you take adds up, and your pedometer will show it to you.

    So that is it. Just lose the weight, keep active, and you will be a new person. It is that simple...in theory.

Chapter 9

Why We Look Like a Food Pyramid

Losing weight should be simple. Just follow a recommended diet, and the weight should fly off. However, there are well over 2,000 different diets to choose from. So who is right? Basically there are about 8 diets that stand alone with many variations. I would like to explore the most popular.

No one can deny that the traditional USDA food pyramid has influenced more people than any other diet. It was developed in the late 1950s-60s when physicians and nutritionists noted a significant rise in the risk of heart disease in those who ate a high fat diet as compared to those who ate a low fat diet.

Much research was done and the now very familiar food pyramid that follows was developed.

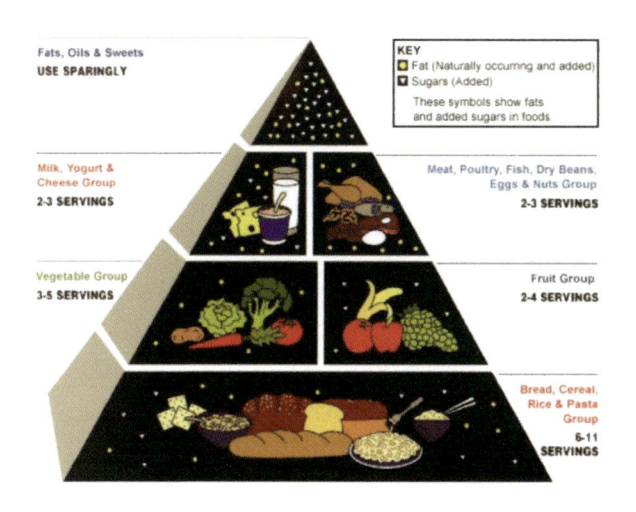

http://illuminations.nctm.org

We all recognize it because it was taught in school and appeared on nearly every cereal box in America. The premise was simple: we eat too much fat, so let's reduce the fat content and replace it with carbohydrate. While in itself this is not a bad idea, the problem becomes one of partial education and the business of selling food products. Education on moving to a high carbohydrate, low fat diet was not followed up with clear education on how much a portion should be. In 1950 people ate small portions, and it was assumed this would follow with the new pyramid. The unintended consequence was twofold. First, a higher fat diet causes much more satiety (sense of fullness), and smaller portions are eaten. People switching to a high carbohydrate, low fat diet will need more carbohydrate to get the same sense of satiety.

The second consequence was that at the time this diet was introduced we Americans were entering a food revolution. Because of advances in farming and food production, for the first time in history it was cheap to produce food. Competition increased as more and more manufacturers entered the food market, both in retail and restaurant sales. This led to two important results for the consumer: lower prices and larger portions to attract more business. The result was that we ate more - more carbohydrate, more fat, and more protein. However, we ate fewer fruits and fresh vegetables as manufacturers made it cheaper to prepare Hamburger Helper rather than minute steak and mixed vegetables. And it tasted good. Manufacturers learned that by manipulating fat, sugar, and salt content in foods, people bought more and ate more. They also gained weight. We all thought we were doing what we were supposed to be doing - eating low fat. But we were missing the point. The end result is that the traditional food pyramid did its job: Americans were starting to look like pyramids, narrow at the top and wide at the bottom.

The health care industry took note. Americans were doing a little better with heart disease, but in the early 1980s obesity and diabetes type II (adult onset) were on the rise.

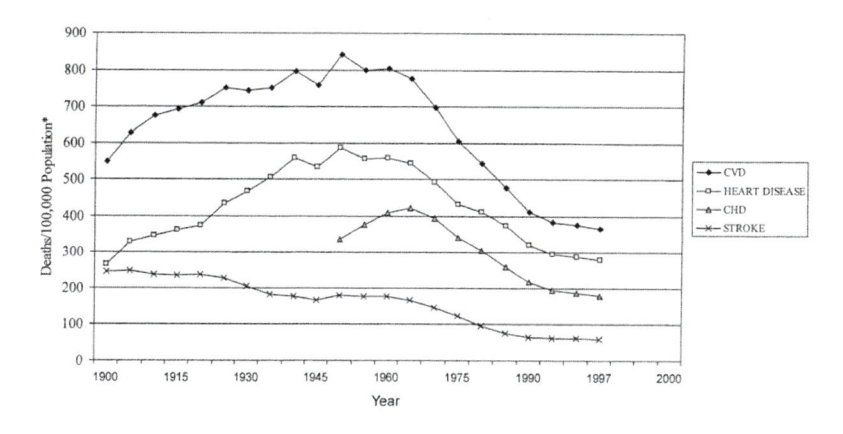

http://www.workhealth.org

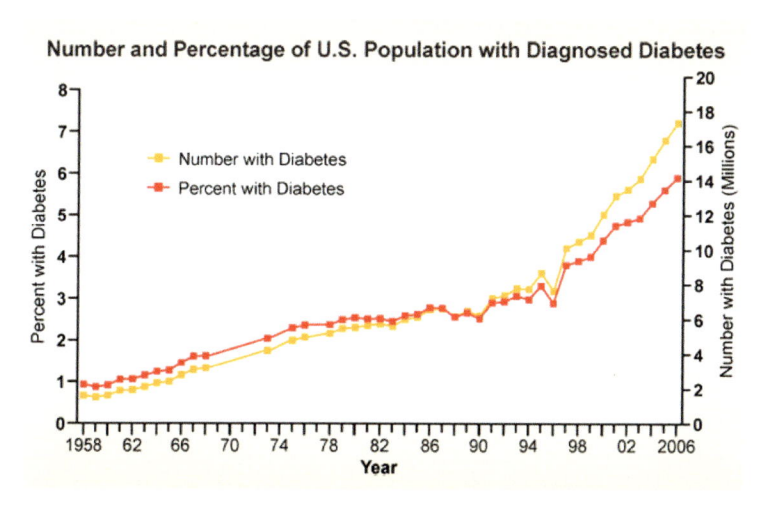

Centers for Disease Control and Prevention. National diabetes fact sheet: general information and national estimates on diabetes in the United States, 2007. Atlanta, GA: U.S. Department of Health and Human Services, Centers for Disease Control and Prevention, 2008.
Division of Health and Nutrition Examination Surveys

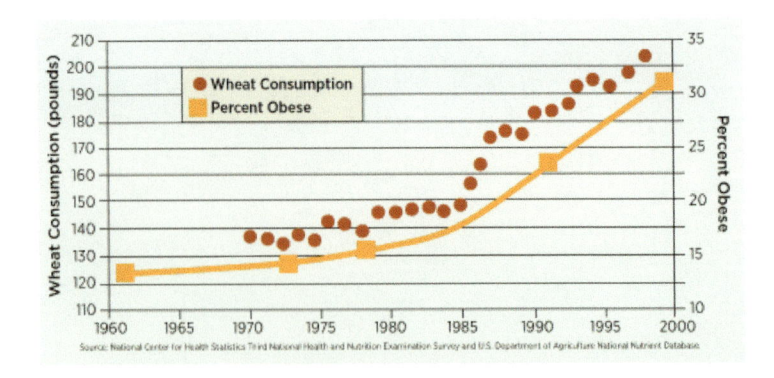

http://profile.prevention.com

At about this time, the Mayo Clinic realized that the new American diet was not the answer to heart disease but a source of a whole new set of chronic diseases spurred on by obesity and its consequences. Research was conducted at Mayo, and they were the first to recommend a change in American nutrition, the Mayo Diet.

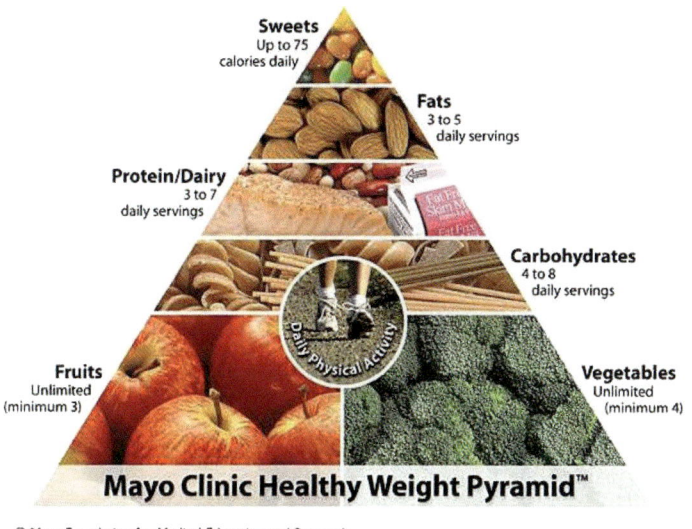

http://www.balancedweightmanagement.com

At the time the Mayo Diet was published, I was in medical residency and we all thought this was the breakthrough Americans needed to reduce the consequences of obesity. This diet stressed the importance of fresh vegetables and fruit more than carbohydrates while still maintaining a low fat approach. Exercise was integrated into the Mayo Diet, yet the diet never really caught on. This was because the USDA was working on a new diet pyramid that would address not just obesity but the significant lack of calcium intake the typical American diet fostered.

We all recognize the new diet as the new food pyramid seen on the following page:

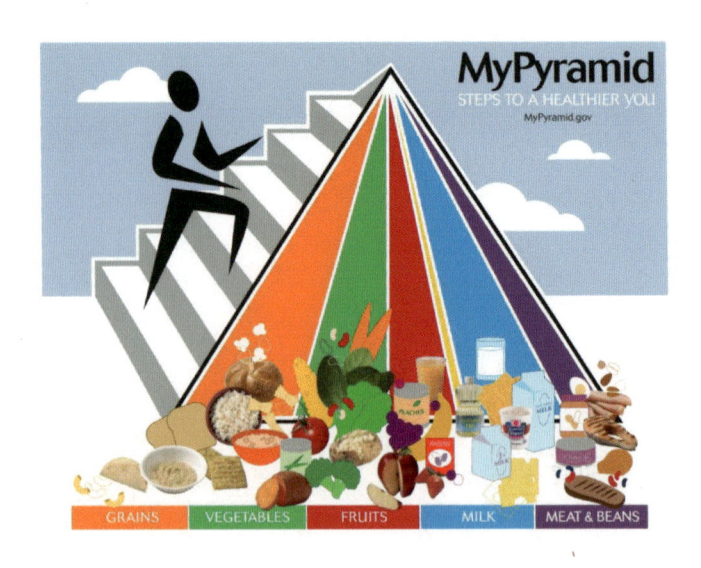

http://justfacs.com

    The first thing to notice in the new pyramid is that exercise is a vital part of good health. Unfortunately, the chart shows a figure running up stairs. Stairs happen to be one of the most avoided exercises and are more likely to turn people off than inspire them. Stairs give the impression that one needs really vigorous exercise for it to mean anything. This is far from the truth. Just about anything other than watching TV counts as exercise.

    The second point is that the new food pyramid embodies our politically correct culture. You will notice that there is no hierarchy of foods. Grains are just as important as milk, beans, and vegetables. A small sliver of fat lies between fruits and milk, but sweets are gone and no longer considered part of a healthy diet.

    One thing I like about the new food pyramid is that

people can go on line to myfoodpyramid.gov and enter their own data to get a personalized evaluation of their nutrition and compare it to the new food pyramid standards. So what's not to like? The new food pyramid's biggest concern is that the USDA did notice that people, particularly girls ages 11-25, are not getting enough calcium in their diets. The new pyramid addresses this by making dairy a very prominent part of the daily diet. "Get your three a day," as the saying goes. However, in order for this to happen and still maintain the needed protein and grains from previous recommendations, the USDA reduced meat servings, added beans, and assumed people would get the rest of their protein from dairy products. I encourage you to test this new food pyramid yourself. You will have a hard time matching up to their standards. It is just not easy.

As I look at these two food pyramids I see the politics of health care shining through. I see the old food pyramid responding to problems in a high fat diet and developing a food pyramid rich in low fat grains. I think of it as the "General Mills diet." While this helped lead America to an obesity epidemic (high fructose corn syrup is another large factor), the USDA saw the error in its ways and with new research found people were not getting enough calcium. The pyramid was revamped, and now I see the new food pyramid as the "American Dairy Association diet."

The idea was okay. However, major reasons girls in

their teens are low in calcium are twofold. First, they are very concerned with their weight and appearance. Girls think drinking too much milk makes them fat because it has lots of calories (in reality, not that many, but we are talking about teen girls). So to keep their weight down, they switch to diet sodas. Now they drink zero calories and look cool and are happy and boys love them, or at least that's what commercials say. The problem with soda is that it has phosphorous in it. Calcium and phosphorous need to be balanced within our bodies. If we increase phosphorous intake, our bodies will remove calcium from our bones to balance the intake. If one does not ingest calcium then the bones suffer. For females ages 11 to 25, this is when the majority of bone deposition occurs. These are also the peak ages of diet soda consumption. So the new food pyramid makes some sense. It is a solid diet, but if you are obese you will find it very difficult to lose weight on this diet because of the glycemic index it possesses.

  Another very popular diet is the Ornish Diet. This diet is more similar to the traditional food pyramid. The Ornish Diet, however, focuses on whole grains as a mainstay. The use of red meats and fats is very limited. This diet does reduce heart disease because of its use of healthy fats and low saturated fats. Dr. Ornish has had excellent success in his laboratory with rats living to a very old age on this diet. Unfortunately, with poor compliance the diet loses all of its beneficial effects.

The Mediterranean Diet is another diet rich in whole grains, seafood, and limited saturated fats and red meats. Statistics show that people who live in the Mediterranean region enjoy very long life with low levels of heart disease. This diet also espouses the use of red wines to enhance antioxidant effects. The diet appeals to most people because it is a very flavorful, rich diet. Unfortunately, the use of this diet does not necessarily extend the benefits that people living in the Mediterranean region enjoy. Genetics are certainly a factor in these people's low risk for heart disease. People of the Mediterranean also enjoy a significantly higher level of exercise than those in America, based on the topography and lifestyle of their cities.

Two diets in response to the USDA pyramids and the study on glycemic index are the South Beach Diet and the Zone Diet. As we've discussed, in 1981 Dr. David Jenkins was a pioneer in glycemic index of foods. He and his colleagues were the first to study the relationship between foods eaten and blood sugar response. He went on to rate foods by their glycemic index. While his concern was for the diabetic patient and the post-gastric bypass patient who suffered from post-meal hypoglycemia secondary to insulin response, it became apparent that normal subjects could also benefit from food ratings.

After several more years of research the South Beach and Zone diets were developed and have been very popular.

Both of these diets recognize the idea that foods are drugs in the sense that depending on your food choice and dose (portion size), the body will respond differently. Thus, if one eats a low glycemic diet, the uneven rises and dips in blood sugar and insulin can be avoided and a lower total calorie diet can be consumed without the hunger associated with eating a low calorie food pyramid or new food pyramid diet.

Dr. Robert Atkins took it a little further. He postulated that if some is good, more is better. The goal of the Atkins Diet was to be very low carbohydrate. While the American Diabetic Association recommended 45-65 grams of carbohydrate per meal, the Atkins Diet recommended total daily carbohydrates of less than 20 grams. He had excellent results. The goal was to develop a state of ketosis. When our bodies are no longer burning a significant portion of calories in glucose and we convert to fat burning, we reduce the spent fats to ketones. This can be measured in the urine and checked by the dieter for compliance.

The Atkins Diet did do well. Unfortunately, when people went off the diet approximately 97% had significant weight regain. I suspect this was mostly because of the preponderance of high carbohydrate food options available in America, and the subjects who responded so well to the Atkins Diet were also the ones most susceptible to weight gain with a high carbohydrate diet.

Probably the most successful early example of an

Atkins style diet was the Lewis and Clark Corps of Discovery in 1803. Over a three-year period, these gentlemen traveled up the Missouri River, over the Bitterroot Mountains, and down the Columbia River and back. They worked very hard at this, and it is estimated they burned 12,000 calories a day. Their diet consisted of whatever they could shoot, pick, or dig. What little grain they had in their diet was eaten early in the expedition. One man died early on from appendicitis. The rest of the Corps survived quite well on an Atkins style diet. Only when they were in the Bitterroot Mountains did they suffer significantly. However, this was due to the fact that there was no food, not its consistency. Native Americans were an important element in their success by giving them high protein foods and leading them through their journey. The natives were not farmers and were also on a low glycemic diet.

As you probably suspect, I am a fan of the Corps of Discovery and have been on parts of the Trail of Discovery. However, while Lewis and Clark were forced into eating a high protein, low carbohydrate diet, the trail today is filled with fast food alternatives that would make their heads spin. Some will even say that if Lewis and Clark were to travel their route again today and live off current offerings as they did then, they would have heart attacks and diabetes before they reached the Pacific Ocean.

Chapter 10
The Measuring Cup Free Diet

Over my years of clinical experience in bariatric medicine I have come to realize that dieting should not be a complicated process. The Boy Scouts use a phrase, "Keep It Simple, Stupid." The KISS principal should also be applied to one's eating habits.

After personal experimentation I devised a very simple diet based on body size that would work for every person. This makes calorie counting obsolete because portions are controlled by the size of your hand. Thus, your measuring cup, your hand, will be proportional to your lean body mass. However, before starting on this diet, there are several supplements I recommend. The first is water intake. The daily recommendation of water intake is 64 ounces a day. This amounts to eight 8-ounce glasses of water daily. Your urine will tell you if you've had enough water. If you are hydrated, your urine should appear fairly clear in the toilet. If your urine is dark yellow, you are not drinking enough and need to increase your water intake. Common reasons to increase water intake are heavy exercise, hot sweaty days in summer, and cold dry days in winter. Some studies show that one does not need to drink extra water to lose weight. However, this is not why I recommend plenty of fluids. Obese people tend to confuse hunger with thirst. When we are young we know when we are thirsty, but over the years we get confused. We find that by eating foods, particularly carbohydrates, we quench our thirst because sugars are burned and become water and carbon dioxide. Thus, over time as we slake our thirst, we associate thirst with hunger. By drinking plenty of fluids thirst is eliminated, limiting our sense of hunger and reducing one trigger for eating.

I also recommend that patients starting a diet program take a generic multivitamin. Multivitamins are available over the counter, and most contain 100% of recommended vitamins and minerals. When working with weight loss, three elements become essential: selenium, chromium, and iodine. If your multivitamin contains these elements it will likely contain all of the other essential vitamins and minerals. Medically, if you eat a healthy diet you do not need to take a multivitamin. However, 90% of an American's food has been grown on the same 10% of the land for the last 40 years. Many of the micronutrients that were once available in the soil have been depleted through this farming practice. It is a small insurance policy to take a multivitamin to counteract this deficiency.

Vitamin D has become a hot topic in nutrition in the last few years. The only known disease caused by lack of vitamin D is chondromalacia, better known as rickets. This disease causes diffuse bone aches and pains along with bone deformity. Recent research has discovered that women who are low in vitamin D and have breast cancer have a worse prognosis than women with normal vitamin D levels. This was also found to be true in cases of ovarian cancer and uterine cancer. Research indicates this trend continues in both men and women with colon cancer, heart disease, and diabetes. It has also been determined that vitamin D deficiency in bariatric patients causes a much slower weight loss. In my practice I have found that supplementing vitamin D in patients who are low in vitamin D leads to a better sense of well-being for most patients and definitely improved weight loss.

In regard to that sense of well-being, seasonal affective disorder (SAD) is a condition seen mostly in northern climates where the winter days are short and the nights are long. People become depressed and grumpy. We treat it with high intensity lamps called Lux lights to simulate a more intense sun exposure. I personally do not have SAD. I just know my wife is much harder to live with in the winter. She thinks I do have SAD. She even gave me Lux lights for Christmas. They do work. She became nice and much easier to get along with. After I leaned about vitamin D and started supplementing my diet, I found I didn't need the lights as much. Just by my taking vitamin D, my wife was nicer all winter long and my appetite easier to control. While I am not saying SAD is caused by vitamin D deficiency, treating vitamin D deficiency may improve mood and be a factor in SAD.

The next supplement I recommend to bariatric patients

is omega-3 fatty acid. Most patients take this in the form of 1200 mg of fish oil once daily. There is ongoing research as to the proper dose of fish oil. For the average patient interested in weight loss, 1200 mg to 3600 mg should be fine. Fish oil has been found to enhance weight loss and reduce triglycerides and insulin levels.

There are certain nutrients we need every day to maintain metabolic function: protein, vitamins, minerals, fats, and fiber. To design a weight loss diet these must be accounted for and still maintain a negative calorie balance. By taking good points from other diets and making it simple to follow, I have devised what I like to call a Measuring Cup Free Diet. The principals are simple. What do we need in a daily diet and what can we live without?

An issue I have with much of the dietary advice given to people these days is that portions are generalized to everyone. It is clear that a 6-foot, 5-inch man has different nutritional needs than a 5-foot, 2-inch woman. Yet, we are bombarded with set portion sizes for all. This cannot work in a successful weight reduction program. There has to be a simple way to judge what a proper portion should be for each individual.

I enjoy astronomy. It is a beautiful hobby that can be enjoyed day and night from your armchair to the North Pole and everywhere in between. One of the first steps in astronomy is getting one's bearings in the night sky. We do this by learning landmark stars and patterns in the sky and using them to "star hop" to new things. Just about everyone recognizes the Big Dipper. It is part of a constellation called Ursa Major or the Great Bear. The tip of the bowl points to the North Star and the handle arcs to Arcturus, a bright star in Bootes as shown below.

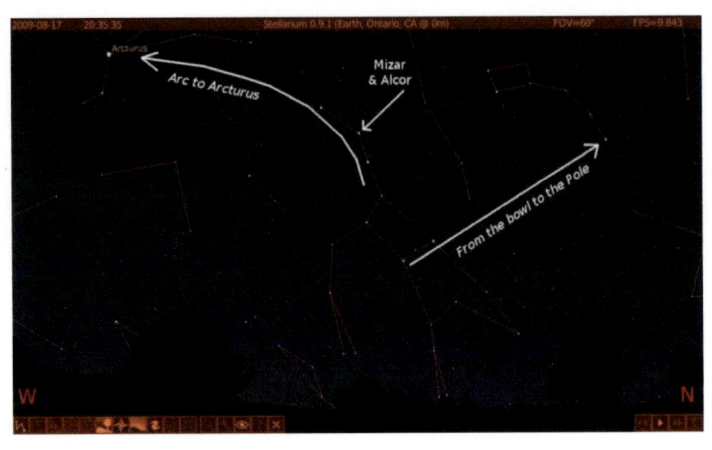

10minuteastronomy.wordpress.com

When star hopping, one has to be able to gauge distances. We use our hands to estimate these distances. If you spread your fingers out and hold your hand at arm's length, the distance from your little finger to your thumb will measure about 25 degrees of the night sky or about the distance across the Big Dipper. Regardless of your size, it will always appear to you to be 25 degrees of night sky. This is because the skeleton is proportional for all people. Thus, the distance between one's eyes is proportional to the length of the arm and hand regardless of height.

Some simple astronomy hand scales are shown on the below.

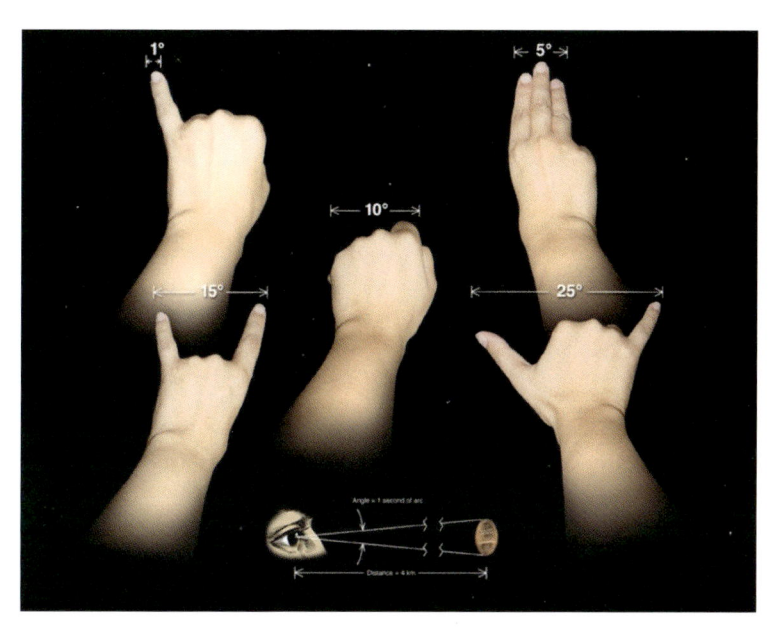

http://chandra.harvard.edu/resources/illustrations/scales.html

I tell you this because it dawned on me one night that the problem with most diets is that a portion for me is not the same as one for my wife or my kids or the other guys in my astronomy club. The proportion of our hands relative to our body size is proportional to our dietary needs.

This is my key to keeping it simple. If you are like me, when you go to a restaurant you assume you will be served the portion that you should eat. However, we all know one will not maintain a reasonable weight on a restaurant diet. But, since we bring our hands to every meal, we can tell how much we need to eat based on our own hands.

So how does it work?

On the next page is an outline of the Measuring Cup Free Diet:

The Measuring Cup Free Diet

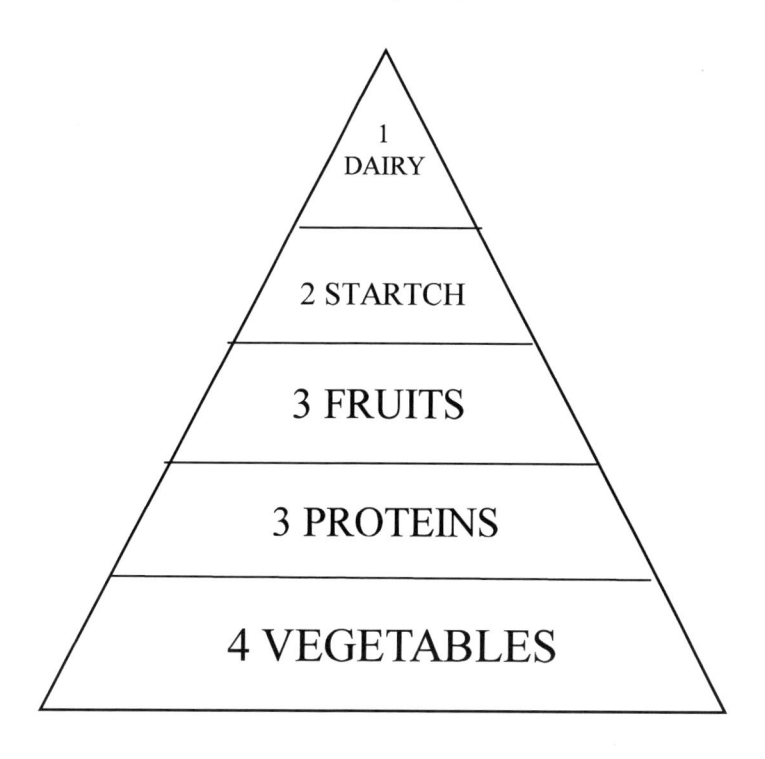

```
        /\
       /1 \
      /DAIRY\
     /--------\
    / 2 STARTCH \
   /--------------\
  /   3 FRUITS     \
 /--------------------\
/    3 PROTEINS        \
--------------------------
/     4 VEGETABLES        \
----------------------------
```

Dairy – 1
1 serving = 8 ounces low fat milk or yogurt, 1/3 c cottage cheese or 1 slice of cheese

Starch - 2
1 serving = 1/3 cup uncooked rice/pasta or ½ potato or 1 slice bread or 1 serving cereal

Fruit – 3
1 serving = kiwi size or 1 c berries or melons

Protein – 3
1 serving = palm size of red meat or palm plus first knuckle of fish/poultry or 3 eggs

Vegetables - 4
1 serving = 2 cupped handfuls of RAW or 1 cupped handful COOKED

Vegetables

In this simple diet one needs 4 servings of vegetables a day. One raw serving of vegetables is measured by cupping your hands as below:

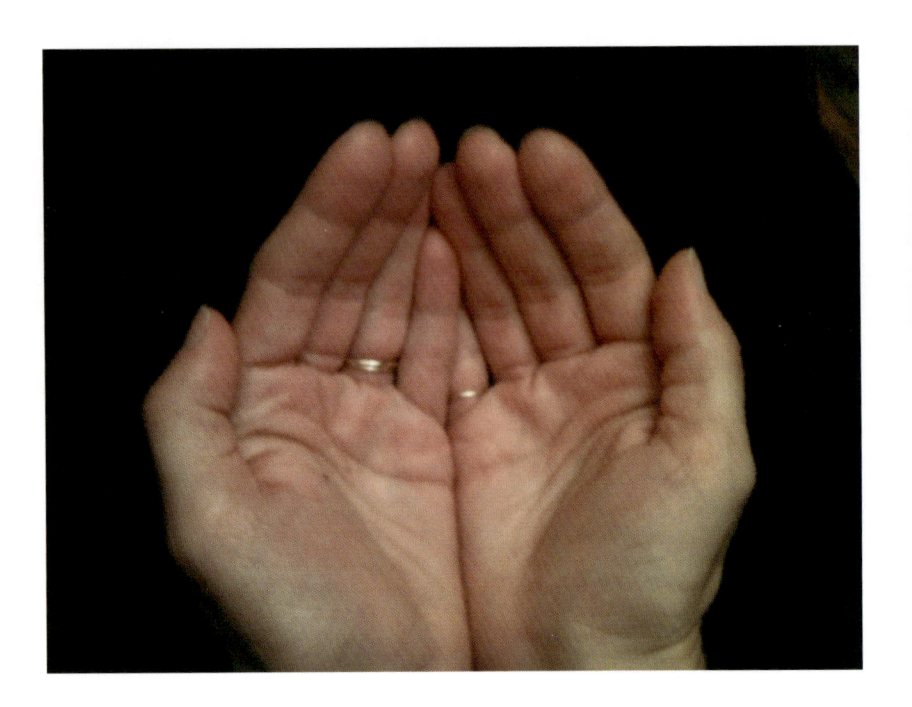

Cooked vegetables will be about half this size. (If you've ever made stir fry, you know that veggies shrink with cooking.)

As a physician I recommend eating a wide variety of vegetables. I do know that many of my bariatric patients are not big vegetable eaters. In fact, rarely do I need to oversee weight loss with people who love vegetables.

A wide variety of food is the spice of life and source of complete nutrition. However, if all you like is ice berg lettuce, then you need four servings a day. Realizing that it may be a struggle to get a variety of vegetables when starting, I compensate poor variety by the use of that multivitamin. The multivitamin does what a limited diet cannot do and provides the vitamins and minerals our bodies need when we do not get them in our foods.

Another great way of getting a variety of vegetables is by using a juicing machine. These handy specialized blenders shred vegetables and fruits, spinning the hard fiber away leaving only the plant's nutritional juice and soluble fiber for you to drink. Many juicers are on the market, and a good one can be had for about $100. Juicing can be a fun way to get a wide variety of vegetables that you might not otherwise eat.

In my practice I have found that many people just do not have much imagination when it comes to vegetables, so here is a list of good vegetable choices:

Vegetable Suggestions:

Asparagus	Broccoli
Artichokes	Brussels sprouts
Bamboo shoots	Cabbage
Beans (green or yellow)	Carrots
Beets	Cauliflower

Celery, celery leaves	Peppers (green, red, sweet, hot)
Chard	
Cucumbers	Radishes
Eggplant	Sauerkraut
Leeks	Spinach
Lettuce	Sprouts
Mushrooms	Summer squash
Okra	Tomatoes
Onions, scallions	Turnips
Pea pods	Zucchini

Source: www.About.com

At this point we need to talk about condiments. Please eat what you like in moderation. Have regular dressing on your salad. Eat ketchup or steak sauce if you need to. If you are doing well with weight loss and enjoying your food, you will have more long term success. If you are doing everything else right and not losing weight, then you must use low fat condiments and limit the quantities. I have found that people who use regular salad dressing eat less and feel more satisfied after eating than those who use low fat dressings. The fat is much more satiating, and less is needed for taste. Understanding these characteristics is what is needed to maintain eating habits that will last a lifetime. It is not enough to lose extra weight; the goal is to keep it off.

Protein

Protein is the most important nutrient to consume in a weight loss program. New research has shown the amino acid leucine, a branched chain amino acid, must be consumed at a level of about 2.5 grams per meal to promote protein synthesis. This equates to a minimum of 30 grams protein per meal. For reasons not fully understood, leucine supplementation does not work. Eating 30 grams of protein leads to a feeling of fullness and muscle synthesis that lasts up to three hours. Most Americans only eat about 10 gms protein for breakfast, 20 for lunch and 60 gms for dinner. By combining at least 30 gms of protein per meal with a low-carbohydrate diet, muscle metabolism is energized, body fat is reduced, and our bodies regulate blood glucose more efficiently.

To give a sense of size, a serving of red meat is about the size of your palm, both in width and depth. A serving of white meat is about the size of your palm and up to the first knuckle. A handful of nuts is a serving of protein. This covers the simplest forms of protein in our diet. Foods such as eggs and legumes are a little trickier and require a little memorizing. Three eggs are one serving. Legumes and beans come out to about a cup. The trouble with beans and legumes is that they contain a fair amount of starch. I have had plenty of patients struggling to lose weight doing everything right, but when we look at their sources of protein and add up total carbohydrates, they are much higher than they should be. This keeps their insulin levels higher. The insulin inhibits the breakdown of fat tissue, and they retain weight. A modification to lower starch protein is usually all that is needed to get the fat to come off.

Eating 30 grams protein per meal is a minimum for all. Based on your body mass, you may need more than 90 grams of protein daily. I recommend eating about 1.5 grams per kilogram of lean body weight. In my practice lean body weight is determined through a body composition scale and measured through electrical impedance. From ehow.com (one of my favorite sites for learning all kinds of things) you can obtain a mathematical method:

1. Weight in pounds
2. Measure waist circumference at the navel
3. Use this formula to calculate percent body fat:

For Women:
[(4.15 x waist measurement) - (0.082 x weight) - 76.76] / weight

For Men:
[(4.15 x waist measurement) - (0.082 x weight) - 98.42] / weight

4. Subtract this number from 100, and this is percent lean body mass

5. Multiply the percent lean mass by your total weight

6. Divide by 2.2 and you have Lean Body Weight in kilograms

This method works, but it is also why I purchased a body composition scale.

If your final value is more than 90, then you need that much protein daily. If your value is less than 90, then you should have 30 grams per meal. You can use this list of protein content of foods to calculate total protein intake. What you will notice is that getting 30 grams of protein may be a struggle. For example: To have a 30 gram breakfast would take 3 eggs, 2 slices of bacon and a cup of low fat yogurt. It is hard to believe that by eating this much for breakfast one can lose weight, but after some trial you will notice it is hard to lose weight and not eat this much.

High-Protein Foods

Beef:

- Hamburger patty, 4 oz = 28 grams protein
- Steak, 6 oz = 42 grams
- Most cuts of beef = 7 grams of protein per ounce

Chicken:

- Chicken breast, 3.5 oz = 30 grams protein
- Chicken thigh = 10 grams (for average size)
- Drumstick = 11 grams
- Wing = 6 grams
- Chicken meat, cooked, 4 oz = 35 grams

Fish:

- Most fish fillets or steaks contain about 22 grams of protein for 3.5 oz (100 grams) of cooked fish, or 6 grams per ounce
- Tuna, 6 oz can = 40 grams of protein

Pork:

- Pork chop, average = 22 grams protein
- Pork loin or tenderloin, 4 oz = 29 grams
- Ham, 3 oz serving = 19 grams
- Ground pork, 1 oz raw = 5 grams, 3 oz cooked = 22 grams
- Bacon, 1 slice = 3 grams
- Canadian-style bacon (back bacon), slice = 5-6 grams

Eggs and Dairy:

- Egg, large = 6 grams protein

- Milk, 1 cup = 8 grams
- Cottage cheese, ½ cup = 15 grams
- Yogurt, 1 cup = usually 8-12 grams (check label)
- Soft cheeses (Mozzarella, Brie, Camembert) = 6 grams per oz
- Medium cheeses (Cheddar, Swiss) = 7-8 grams per oz
- Hard cheeses (Parmesan) = 10 grams per oz

Beans (including soy):
- Tofu, ½ cup = 20 grams protein
- Tofu, 1 oz = 2.3 grams
- Soy milk, 1 cup = 6-10 grams
- Most beans (black, pinto, lentils, etc) = about 7-10 grams protein per half cup of cooked beans
- Soy beans, ½ cup cooked = 14 grams protein
- Split peas, ½ cup cooked = 8 grams

Nuts and Seeds:
- Peanut butter, 2 tablespoons = 8 grams protein
- Almonds, ¼ cup = 8 grams
- Peanuts, ¼ cup = 9 grams
- Cashews, ¼ cup = 5 grams
- Pecans, ¼ cup = 2.5 grams
- Sunflower seeds, ¼ cup = 6 grams

- Pumpkin seeds, ¼ cup = 8 grams
- Flax seeds, ¼ cup = 8 grams

Source: www.About.com

Fruit

Next on the pyramid is fruit. In the Measuring Cup Free Diet a serving of fruit is defined by the size of a kiwi. It has the right density and feel. The next time you go to the grocery store, buy a kiwi and get a good feel of its size and weight. Compare it to other fruits. You will notice that a banana is about equal to two kiwis. Thus, a banana is two servings. A small apple is one, as is a small orange, half of a grapefruit, and so on. For the fruits that are hard to measure such as blueberries, melons, and strawberries, it comes out to about one cup per serving.

One serving of fruit juice is four ounces. If you want juice for your fruit, please do not use juice from concentrate. I do not promote substituting juice for your fruit servings because you miss out on one very important part of the fruit, and that is fiber. The older you get, the more you realize how important fiber is to a diet.

Vegetables, protein, and fruit are the most important parts of a well-balanced diet. We need them for everything our body does. Do not skip them! Regardless of the future of your eating habits, eat your veggies, protein, and fruits. To lose weight, therefore, we need to cut calories from somewhere. Since we need the vegetables, protein, and fruit, we must reduce starch and dairy. This works out great, because you can survive without them in your diet.

Starch

I limit starches to two servings a day during weight loss for two reasons. First, this limits calories. Second, starch causes a significant rise in blood sugar that in turn causes most of us with a weight problem to release too much insulin and limit fat burning even in a low calorie state. The irony for many of us is that we crave starch. It tastes so good and gives us the buzz of the sugar rush. Comfort food equals happy feelings. It is the yin and yang of life. But the foods that give us so much comfort make us feel so uncomfortable.

So what are they?

Carbohydrates

Bread	Pasta
Cereals	Corn
Rice	Potatoes

Corn and potatoes are not counted as vegetables because of their starch content. This is unfortunate because they are the sole source of vegetables for many Americans. We eat a lot of them.

One slice of bread is one serving of the bread and

cereals category. (Not one of those 400-grain breads that weigh 12 ounces each slice.) I'm saying one slice of medium grain wheat bread is one serving by weight. For cereals, if it weighs as much as a slice of bread, it is one serving. This comes out to about a quarter cup of oatmeal (uncooked) or about ¾ cup Rice Krispies. I am not worried about exact science. Just keep the cereal portions close to the weight of a slice of wheat bread. This takes into account calorie density and gives a simple measure of carbohydrate content.

Rice can be measured raw at 1/3 cup or cooked at 1 cup. Pasta is the same. If you weigh a third of a cup of rice or pasta, you will see it weighs about as much as a slice of wheat bread. Again, it is all about calorie density.

A serving of corn is ½ cup and for potatoes it is ½ of a small baked potato. These veggies are starchy and well hydrated, so they do not measure against bread.

Dairy

At the peak of the pyramid is dairy. To keep the calorie count down while allowing for adequate protein and fruits and vegetables, we must limit dairy. As a result of excellent advertising by the American Dairy Association, we as Americans have been conditioned to make sure we get our dairy. We do not actually need dairy in a balanced diet. In fact, we as a species did not consume dairy (after being weaned) for the first 90,000 years of our existence. It is only since the advent of farming that non-human milk was introduced into our diet. Dairy is a good source of nutrition but difficult to use in weight loss because of its lower protein value compared to its sugar (lactose) content. One eight-ounce serving of skim milk, one cup of low fat yogurt, 1/3 cup cottage cheese, or one slice of any other cheese is the dairy allowance for the day. You will be consuming a calcium/vitamin D supplement 2 times a day to guarantee adequate calcium for bone health.

One of the most important and difficult things to do to lose weight is to keep track of all food and drink. By writing down all that goes into your mouth you accomplish two things. First, if you write down your foods as you eat them, you become mindful of what you are eating. It is much harder to intentionally keep a running tally of 5 Oreo cookies after a hard day at work than it is to have a binge and hours later reflect back over the day and recall what was eaten.

Secondly, when you find yourself hungry or up in weight and you do not know why, being able to look back over the last 1-3 days can provide the clue. Often patients develop a pattern I call carbohydrate cycling. It usually starts with a high starch meal such as pizza or a breakfast of toast and oatmeal. Blood sugars rise and insulin is released. A few hours later hunger sets in as blood sugar drops. As habits take over, another carbohydrate rich meal usually follows. Many times protein intake goes down, and the cycle begins. If left unchecked, after a couple of days the fat-burning enzymes that were built up quickly diminish, and now the patient is no longer burning fat but making fat. To stop the cycle one has to void simple carbohydrates from the diet for 4-5 days and go through that uncomfortable hunger phase to rebuild fat-burning enzymes back up to good fat losing levels.

Two other reasons people will suddenly gain weight are alcohol consumption and excessive salt intake. Alcohol and weight loss are not good companions. Alcohol is metabolized to fat and sugar. More importantly, alcohol can cloud our judgment and allow us to eat the foods we would otherwise avoid. This can lead to carbohydrate cycling, frustration, and a sense of hopelessness.

Salt causes water retention. If you have a high salt meal, drink plenty of water over the next few days. This will drive the salt out of your system. It seems counter-intuitive to drink more water when retaining water, but your kidneys will use the salt to rid your body of the excess water intake.

That is the simplicity of the Measuring Cup Free Diet. Everywhere you go you have all that you need to figure out what to eat to lose weight and keep it off. This eating plan is for weight loss.

But what do you do once you are at goal? To maintain your new weight, we need to add back calories. This is done once a week with either a serving of dairy or starch; you decide. Every week add in another serving until you get to the point where your weight loss stops or your weight begins to increase. You may find that you can have two dairy a day or maybe six. It will depend on your metabolism, your food choices, and your activity level. Remember, you must be more active to maintain your weight or you will regain. Do not forget this or your scale will remind you.

Chapter 11
Metabolic Syndrome Work-up

This booklet was designed for use with the two-hour lecture I give for my bariatric weight loss practice. As a physician, I watch for the diseases of fat. The following discusses the laboratory work-up I do on my patients. If you are reading for your own personal benefit, you can stop now, but you may find this interesting nonetheless.

As a bariatrician, I am treating not just obesity. Rather, I am looking to reduce a patient's risk and complications of diseases such as diabetes, heart attack, and stroke and to treat diseases already manifest such as NASH (fat-induced liver disease) and sleep apnea. The laboratory workup I do gives me a snap-shot of a patient's bariatric health.

First I look at the CBC or complete blood count. This lab is a misnomer for the lay public, because it is not a complete blood evaluation but an evaluation of the red and white blood cells. This gives clues to nutritional problems such as anemia (low iron) and vitamin B complex deficiencies. If abnormalities are found, I add further labs as indicated.

Next I check kidney functions. Obesity is as hard on the kidneys as fasting. Knowing what salts are in the blood and how well the kidneys are doing is important. Many of the diseases related to obesity affect the kidneys also, such as hypertension and diabetes. I also check a magnesium level because a low level combined with the rapid water loss seen early in weight loss can lead to cramping of muscles, which is quite uncomfortable and preventable. A uric acid level is also checked because obese people are not only more likely to suffer from gout, but weight loss can contribute to a gouty flare.

A C-reactive protein or CRP is checked. This is a non-specific test for inflammation. Obesity, particularly abdominal obesity, can be very inflammatory. This is one reason obesity affects so many other disease processes. If the CRP is elevated, it is followed up at 10% weight loss. If not reduced by then, I look for other reasons for the elevation. Because it is a non-specific test, it may not be elevated due to visceral fat, and another cause should be found.

I also run a complete lipid profile. This consists of the total cholesterol, triglycerides, LDL (bad cholesterol), and HDL (good cholesterol). Obese people tend to have bad cholesterol as I have outlined above and will discuss later with metabolic syndrome.

I do a full thyroid panel as well. Every person who has a weight problem and has seen a doctor thinks at one time or another that it is a "gland problem." So the doctor checks a TSH, finds it in the normal range, and says, "Nope, it's not your glands." But there is now evidence that the patient may be more right than previously thought. To understand this, you have to be able to understand the thyroid test, which can be confusing. The TSH or thyroid stimulating hormone is released from the pituitary in the brain and stimulates the thyroid gland in the neck to make thyroxin, the hormone responsible for setting the metabolic rate of the body like a thermostat. Thyroxin then stimulates the brain to reduce TSH production. Thus, if the TSH is high, the thyroid gland is making less thyroxin than the brain thinks is necessary. If the TSH is low, the brain thinks the thyroid gland is making too much thyroxin. To complicate matters, thyroxin comes in two forms, T3 and T4. T3 is the active form of thyroxin, and the 3 stands for the three iodine atoms on the thyroxin hormone. T4, on the other hand, refers to the storage form of thyroxin and has four iodine atoms on it.

For thyroid hormone to be active, it must be converted from T4 to T3. This happens not in the thyroid gland but in the blood stream. Obesity hormones can interfere with this process and lead to a problem called relative hypothyroidism of obesity. This is characterized by symptoms of hypothyroidism such as low energy, constipation, cold intolerance, and a high normal TSH. Having a relatively high T4 and relatively low T3 also cements the diagnosis. Treatment consists of weight loss and replacing the low T3. Once weight loss is achieved, the thyroid replacement is stopped because the disease process has been fixed through weight loss. Before you get excited, this is not as common as you might hope, and your obesity is not likely from relative hypothyroidism of obesity.

Vitamin D is an important test I check. Where I live in Duluth, MN, we have about a 50% deficiency of vitamin D. In my bariatric population it is closer to 80%. We just do not get as much sun as southern states. And, let's face it, obese people don't run around in the summer with a lot of skin exposed.

Liver functions are another important lab test. Elevated liver tests in obesity are common. Obese people tend to have fatty infiltrated livers. There can be so much fat in the liver that it becomes toxic and causes inflammation of the liver and elevated liver functions. This disease is called NASH or Non-Alcoholic SteatoHepatitis. It is a serious condition of obesity that, if left untreated, can lead to cirrhosis and liver failure and death. Weight loss is the treatment of choice.

An EKG test is also done to evaluate the presence of heart disease and irregular rhythms. Weight loss can put a strain on cardiac function. Knowing the level of heart health is important before recommending an exercise program.

Lastly, I check a urinalysis. A weight loss diet is a stress to the body and confirming good filtering ability of the kidneys is important.

One reason I check these labs is that I am looking for a process called metabolic syndrome. Metabolic syndrome is a constellation of laboratory parameters that if present increases one's risk for diabetes, heart attack, and stroke. There is controversy in the literature as to whether this is a true disease entity or just a compilation of added risks listed separately. Regardless, all agree that metabolic syndrome is a serious issue. To have metabolic syndrome you must have at least three of these five symptoms:

1. Blood pressure of 135/85 or more or be treated for hypertension
2. Fasting blood sugar of 100 mg/dl or more
3. HDL cholesterol under 45 mg/dl for men or under 50 mg/dl for women
4. Triglycerides of 150 mg/dl or more
5. Waist circumference of 40 inches or more for men or 35 inches or more for women   (This is race specific for European Americans. Lower values apply for shorter people such as Southeast Asians = 35.5 inches for men and 31.5 inches for women)

Study this list and you will see that metabolic syndrome

is a disease of insulin resistance and obesity. First, high blood pressure is directly related to fat. Second, elevated blood sugar, low HDL, and triglycerides are insulin effects. And lastly, a larger waist circumference measures visceral fat. All together, metabolic syndrome shows how visceral fat and high insulin levels are metabolically active and devastating for stroke, heart attack, and diabetes type II.

Conclusion

I truly hope that this has been an eye opening insight into the chronic disease of obesity. As a physician, knowing what one is treating is the most important first step to rapid resolution. Unfortunately, obesity is a chronic disease and requires daily treatment by you, the patient. Even the root of the word patient means to carry a burden. What could be more of a burden than the extra weight we carry?

When you are ready, begin your journey. You have the power to start this process, in which you will need to accomplish three goals. First, change the way you relate to food. Food is your drug for obesity. Food has been a drug many have used for years to celebrate the good times and provide comfort in the bad times. It has been a sleep substitute and the warm hug we needed when we were alone. Food has the power to do this. But if used properly, food can be the drug that sets you free from its excessive burden.

Secondly, make activity a cornerstone of your life. The weight loss will come, but only with exercise added will it stay off for a lifetime. It takes two years of diligence before a habit is internalized and part of your being. My brother-in-law is right. It does take will power to lose weight, but it takes perseverance to keep it off. Give yourself two years of activity that you find enjoyable, and it will keep the weight where you want it to be - someone else's problem.

Lastly, you need to give yourself permission. You need permission to start, permission to fail, and, most importantly, permission to accept responsibility and start again. This is a chronic disease requiring a lifetime of treatment. As Yogi Berra said, "It aint over 'til it's over."

Glycemic Index of Common Foods

FOOD	Glycemic index (glucose = 100)	Serving size (grams)	Glycemic load per serving
BAKERY PRODUCTS AND BREADS			
Banana cake, made with sugar	47	60	14
Banana cake, made without sugar	55	60	12
Sponge cake, plain	46	63	17
Vanilla cake made from packet mix with vanilla frosting (Betty Crocker)	42	111	24
Apple, made with sugar	44	60	13
Apple, made without sugar	48	60	9
Waffles, Aunt Jemima (Quaker Oats)	76	35	10
Bagel, white, frozen	72	70	25
Baguette, white, plain	95	30	15
Coarse barley bread, 75-80% kernels, average	34	30	7
Hamburger bun	61	30	9
Kaiser roll	73	30	12
Pumpernickel bread	56	30	7
50% cracked wheat kernel bread	58	30	12
White wheat flour bread	71	30	10
Wonder™ bread, average	73	30	10

Whole wheat bread, average	71	30	9
100% Whole Grain™ bread (Natural Ovens)	51	30	7
Pita bread, white	68	30	10
Corn tortilla	52	50	12
Wheat tortilla	30	50	8
BEVERAGES			
Coca Cola®, average	63	250 mL	16
Fanta®, orange soft drink	68	250 mL	23
Lucozade®, original (sparkling glucose drink)	95±10	250 mL	40
Apple juice, unsweetened, average	44	250 mL	30
Cranberry juice cocktail (Ocean Spray®)	68	250 mL	24
Gatorade	78	250 mL	12
Orange juice, unsweetened	50	250 mL	12
Tomato juice, canned	38	250 mL	4
BREAKFAST CEREALS AND RELATED PRODUCTS			
All-Bran™, average	55	30	12
Coco Pops™, average	77	30	20
Cornflakes™, average	93	30	23
Cream of Wheat™ (Nabisco)	66	250	17
Cream of Wheat™, Instant (Nabisco)	74	250	22
Grapenuts™, average	75	30	16
Muesli, average	66	30	16
Oatmeal, average	55	250	13
Instant oatmeal, average	83	250	30
Puffed wheat, average	80	30	17
Raisin Bran™ (Kellogg's)	61	30	12

Special K™ (Kellogg's)	69	30	14
GRAINS			
Pearled barley, average	28	150	12
Sweet corn on the cob, average	60	150	20
Couscous, average	65	150	9
Quinoa	53	150	13
White rice, average	89	150	43
Quick cooking white basmati	67	150	28
Brown rice, average	50	150	16
Converted, white rice (Uncle Ben's®)	38	150	14
Whole wheat kernels, average	30	50	11
Bulgur, average	48	150	12
COOKIES AND CRACKERS			
Graham crackers	74	25	14
Vanilla wafers	77	25	14
Shortbread	64	25	10
Rice cakes, average	82	25	17
Rye crisps, average	64	25	11
Soda crackers	74	25	12
DAIRY PRODUCTS AND ALTERNATIVES			
Ice cream, regular	57	50	6
Ice cream, premium	38	50	3
Milk, full fat	41	250 mL	5
Milk, skim	32	250 mL	4
Reduced-fat yogurt with fruit, average	33	200	11
FRUITS			
Apple, average	39	120	6
Banana, ripe	62	120	16

Dates, dried	42	60	18
Grapefruit	25	120	3
Grapes, average	59	120	11
Orange, average	40	120	4
Peach, average	42	120	5
Peach, canned in light syrup	40	120	5
Pear, average	38	120	4
Pear, canned in pear juice	43	120	5
Prunes, pitted	29	60	10
Raisins	64	60	28
Watermelon	72	120	4
BEANS AND NUTS			
Baked beans, average	40	150	6
Blackeye peas, average	33	150	10
Black beans	30	150	7
Chickpeas, average	10	150	3
Chickpeas, canned in brine	38	150	9
Navy beans, average	31	150	9
Kidney beans, average	29	150	7
Lentils, average	29	150	5
Soy beans, average	15	150	1
Cashews, salted	27	50	3
Peanuts, average	7	50	0
PASTA and NOODLES			
Fettucini, average	32	180	15
Macaroni, average	47	180	23
Macaroni and Cheese (Kraft)	64	180	32
Spaghetti, white, boiled, average	46	180	22
Spaghetti, white, boiled 20 min, average	58	180	26

Spaghetti, whole meal, boiled, average	42	180	17
SNACK FOODS			
Corn chips, plain, salted, average	42	50	11
Fruit Roll-Ups®	99	30	24
M & M's®, peanut	33	30	6
Microwave popcorn, plain, average	55	20	6
Potato chips, average	51	50	12
Pretzels, oven-baked	83	30	16
Snickers Bar®	51	60	18
VEGETABLES			
Green peas, average	51	80	4
Carrots, average	35	80	2
Parsnips	52	80	4
Baked russet potato, average	111	150	33
Boiled white potato, average	82	150	21
Instant mashed potato, average	87	150	17
Sweet potato, average	70	150	22
Yam, average	54	150	20
MISCELLANEOUS			
Hummus (chickpea salad dip)	6	30	0
Chicken nuggets, frozen, reheated in microwave oven 5 min	46	100	7
Pizza, plain baked dough, served with parmesan cheese and tomato sauce	80	100	22
Pizza, Super Supreme (Pizza Hut)	36	100	9
Honey, average	61	25	12

The complete list of the glycemic index and glycemic load for more than 1,000 foods can be found in the article "International tables of glycemic index and glycemic load values: 2008" by Fiona S. Atkinson, Kaye Foster-Powell, and Jennie C. Brand-Miller in the December 2008 issue of **Diabetes Care**, Vol. 31, number 12, pages 2281-2283.

http://www.health.harvard.edu/newsweek/Glycemic_index_and_glycemic_load_for_100_foods.htm

References

Achievements in public health U.S. 1900-1999, decline in deaths from heart disease and stroke – United States, 1900-1999. Centers for Disease Control. August 6, 1999 / Vol. 48 / No. 30 retrieved 23 April 15, 2013 from publichealthreviews.eu/show/f/.

Adiposopathy – defining, diagnosing, and establishing indications to treat 'sick fat': what are the regulatory considerations? Bays, Harold. *US Endocrine Diaease 2006; Issue 2:12-14*

Calcium and dairy acceleration of weight and fat loss during energy restriction in obese adults Zemel Michael B. , Thompson, Warren, Milstead, Anita, Morris, Kristin and Campbell, Peter *Obesity Research (2004) 12, 582–590*

Comparison of the Atkins, Ornish, Weight Watchers, and Zone Diets for weight loss and heart disease risk reduction: a randomized trial Michael L. Dansinger, MD, Joi Augustin Gleason, MS, RD, John L. Griffith, PhD, Harry P. Selker, MD, MSPH, Ernst J. Schaefer, MD *JAMA. 2005; 293(1):43-5*

Comparison of low fat and low carbohydrate diets on circulating fatty acid composition and markers of inflammation Forsythe CE, et al. *Lipids. 2008 Jan;43(1):65-77. Epub 2007 Nov 29.*

Dietary protein impact on glycemic control during weight loss. Layman DK, Baum Jl. *J. Nutr. 2004; 134:9685-9735.*

A descriptive study of individuals successful at long-term maintenance of substantial weight loss Klem ML, Wing RR, McGuire MT, Seagle HM, Hill JO *Am J Clin Nutr. 1997 Aug; 66(2):239-46.*

Effect of fructose overfeeding and fish oil administration on hepatic de novo lipogenesis and insulin sensitivity in healthy men. Faeh D, Minehira K, Schwarz JM, Periasamy R, Park S, Tappy L.*Diabetes. 2005 Jul; 54(7):1907-13.*

The End of Overeating Taking Control of the Insatiable American Appetite Kessler David A., Rodale Books Emmaus, Pennsylvania, USA.2009. ISBN: 978-1-60529-785-9.

Energy expenditure of nonexercise activity James A Levine, Sara J Schleusner, Michael D Jensen *Am J Clin Nutr December 2000 vol. 72 no. 6 1451-1454*

Handbook of Obesity Eitiology and Pathophysiology Second Edition Bray, George, Bouchard, Clause.

Inadequate sleep as a risk factor for obesity: analyses of the NHANES I. Gangwisch JE, Malaspina D, Boden-Albala B, Heymsfield SB. *Sleep. 2005 Oct; 28(10):1289-96*

In the face of contradictory evidence: Report of the Dietary Guidelines for Americans Committee Adele H. Hite M.A.T. a, Richard David Feinman Ph.D. b,*, Gabriel E. Guzman Ph.D., Morton Satin M.Sc. d, Pamela A. Schoenfeld R.D. e, Richard J. Wood Ph.D. *Nutrition 26 (2010) 915–924*

Lipolysis and the intergrated physiology of lipid energy metabolism Wang,S,K,G, Soni,et al. *MolGenet Metab - 2008 95(3): 117-26*

Metabolic syndrome in a family practice population Prevalence and clinical characteristics Caroline van den Hooven, MSC, Janneke Ploemacher, MSC, and Marshall Godwin, MD, MSC, FCFP *Can Fam Physician. 2006 August 10; 52(8): 983*

National diabetes fact sheet: general information and national estimates on diabetes in the United States, 2007 Centers for Disease Control and Prevention.. Atlanta, GA: U.S. Department of Health and Human Services, Centers for Disease Control and Prevention, 2008

Only One Man Died The Medical Aspects of the Lewis and Clark Expedition Chuinard, Eldon G. *Ye Galleon Press 2002*

Overlapping neuronal circuits in addiction and obesity: evidence of systems pathology Volkow N.D, Wang G.-J, Fowler J.S., Telang F. *Phil. Trans. R. Soc. B. 2008; 363:3191–3200.*

Potential role of sugar (fructose) in the epidemic of hypertension, obesity and the metabolic syndrome, diabetes, kidney disease, and cardiovascular disease Richard J Johnson, et al.
Am J Clin Nutr October 2007 vol. 86 no. 4 899-906

Prevalence of overweight, obesity, and extreme obesity among adults: United States, trends 1960–1962 through 2007–2008 Ogden, Cynthia L., and Carroll, Margaret D., *Division of Health and Nutrition Examination Surveys*

Prospective study of serum selenium concentrations and esophageal and gastric cardia cancer, heart disease, stroke, and total death. Wei WQ, Abnet CC, Qiao YL, Dawsey SM, Dong ZW, Sun XD, Fan JH, Gunter EW, Taylor PR, Mark SD. *Am J Clin Nutr. 2004 Jan; 79(1):80-5*

A randomized trial comparing a very low-carbohydrate diet and a calorie-restricted low-fat diet on body weight and cardiovascular risk factors in healthy women Brehm BJ, Seely RJ, Daniels SR, D'Alessio DA.. *J Clin Endocrinol Metab 88:1617-1623, 2003*

Randomized trial of weight-loss-diets for young adults varying in fish and fish oil content. - Thorsdottir I - *Int J Obes (Lond) - 01-OCT-2007; 31(10): 1560*

Scales and angular measurement Retrieved April 15, 2013 from Harvard-Smithsonian Center for Astrophysics August 19, 2008 *http://chandra.harvard.edu/resources/illustrations/scales.html*

Subclinical thyroid dysfunction: a joint statement on management from the American Association of Clinical Endocrinologists, the American Thyroid Association, and the Endocrine Society. Gharib H, Tuttle RM, Baskin HJ, et al. *J Clin Endocrinol Metab.2005;90:581-58*

Vitamins for chronic disease prevention in adults: scientific review. Fairfield KM, Fletcher RH. *JAMA. 2002 Jun 19; 287(23):3116-26.*

Vitamin D deficiency Holick, Michael F. *N Enl J Med 2007; 357: 266-81*

Wheat Belly: Lose the Wheat, Lose the Weight, and Find Your Path Back to Health Davis, William, Rodale Books New York, USA.2011. ISBN: 978-1-60961-154-5.

CPSIA information can be obtained at www.ICGtesting.com
Printed in the USA
LVIW01n0905100716
495745LV00001B/5